COVID-19 and the Mark of the Beast

What Every Christian Needs to Know about the Fake Vaccine

Mike Stone

Contents

Author contact: mikestone114@yahoo.com

Throughout this book, I refer to the various COVID-19 injections as vaccines.

In reality, they do not meet the medical or legal definition of a vaccine.

Hence, they are not real vaccines, but gene-altering therapies.

I refer to them as vaccines for reasons of clarity for those readers who are not sufficiently red-pilled.

Portions of this book previously appeared in *Reversing the Side Effects of the COVID-19 Vaccine: How to Heal Yourself from Adverse Reactions to the Vaccine and Protect Yourself from Shedding*.

Chapter One

Is Heaven in Your Future?

Are you a Christian (aka a traditional Catholic)?

Are you concerned about the COVID-19 vaccine?

If you answered yes to both questions, then this is a book you should read.

You won't find the information presented here anywhere else. You won't find it in the mainstream news. You won't find it taught in any school. And you certainly won't find it at your local church or from anyone associated with your local church. That much I can absolute guarantee you.

That you're reading this book tells me you want to go to Heaven. I know that because, first, everyone wants to go to Heaven. And, second, because by reading this book it shows that going to Heaven is something you've thought deeply about.

Unlike the sleeping sheeple that populate most of the planet, you've actually taken your quest for Heaven a step further by researching the necessary steps to get there. Good for you.

As someone who also desires to go to Heaven, I'm happy for you. You just might make it. You just might be one of the very few who actually escapes eternal damnation. That will be quite an achievement, because never before in history has it been harder to get to Heaven.

Never before in history has society been so engulfed in sin.

Never before in history has evil stretched its hand so far and wide across the globe.

The sins of Sodom and Gomorrah were confined largely to those two cities. The sins of today are rampant throughout the entire world. A man who was blessed with more wisdom than his words might indicate, once said, "If God doesn't destroy San Francisco, he owes Sodom and Gomorrah an apology."

That was almost fifty years ago. Today, it's not just San Francisco that's mired in sin and lawlessness; it's every city in every country throughout the world. They're all as bad as Sodom and Gomorrah. Worse than Sodom and Gomorrah, because their sins are not just sins of the flesh, but sins of greed, avarice, rage, violence, rioting, looting, abortion, rape and murder.

Bolshevik Russia and Communist China launched levels of hate, murder and genocide in the 20th century that were never before seen in history, but those crimes were largely confined to their own continents. Today, we are facing the possible murder and extermination of over half of the world's population, maybe even more than half.

Heaven has told us that wars are punishment for the sins of man. Today we are facing the initial onslaught of the greatest spectacle of mass murder ever committed in the history of the world. That tells us that man is guiltier of sin today than ever before in history.

Almost everyone that is slated for death over the next three to five years is going to hell.

Are you?

Chapter Two

We Live in a World Gone Mad

Your grandmother, despite all of your protests, insists on taking the jab, becomes deathly ill and blames you for her demise, because you didn't wear a mask the last time you visited her.

When you tell her your mask status has nothing to do with her illness, she screams and cries and tells you not to visit her anymore.

Your sister and her husband delight in sending you videos of their toddler children squirming and crying after being forced to wear masks, while they laugh with glee in the background.

When you tell them they are endangering the health and safety of their own children, they become hysterically irate and threaten to report you to the police as an extremist.

Your beer-drinking brother, who spends his nights and weekends playing video games and watching porn, and who has never had a girlfriend in his life, calls you a "conspiracy theorist" for questioning the safety of the "vaccine."

When you explain to him that the vaccine isn't really a vaccine at all, but a form of gene-altering therapy, he shouts you down and hangs up the phone.

Your mother, who divorced your father years ago in order to "find herself", informs the family that no one, not even her own children, are welcome in her house anymore if they haven't submitted to the jab.

When you show up and attempt to talk sense to her, she screams and slams the door in your face.

Your wife, without your consent or knowledge, sneaks herself and your children off to get jabbed.

When you ask her where she went, she lies and tells you she was shopping. You discover the truth two days later when your daughter develops blood clots and dies.

You wonder, has the world gone mad?

You step out in the street and see nothing but mask-wearing zombies.

You show up at your job and are shunned by your co-workers for not taking the jab. In the break room you see them, huddled in front of the television set, soaking up every word from the lying newscaster's mouth.

Like your family, and like everyone else around the world, none of them knows anyone who has actually died from the alleged virus, but that hasn't stopped them from falling into full panic mode.

You wonder, has the world gone mad?

You talk to the few friends you still have left, the ones who haven't cancelled you due to your refusal to get jabbed. You attempt to explain to them the seriousness of the situation, but they don't want to hear it. All they care about is their annual summer trip to Disneyland, their thrice-annual trip to Las Vegas, or the latest celebrity gossip. All they want is for everything to return to normal.

When you tell them life is never going back to normal, they terminate the conversation and stop returning your phone calls and emails.

You wonder, has the world gone mad?

You wonder, is humanity living under a Satanic spell?

You wonder, do any of us even have a chance, or are we all doomed to succumb to the Beast?

Chapter Three

Is It a Sin to Take the COVID-19 Vaccine?

> "What is mortal sin? It is a great contempt shown to God. God is not capable of pain; but, were he capable of suffering, a single mortal sin would be sufficient to make him die through sorrow."
>
> –St. Alphonsus Ligouri

Is it a sin to take the COVID-19 vaccine?

In a word, yes.

But is it a serious sin; what Catholics call a mortal sin that will condemn one's soul to hell if not confessed?

Again, yes.

At least one of the currently available COVID-19 vaccines uses aborted baby cells in its production, and *all* of them use abortion-derived cell lines in their lab testing. Therefore, anyone who voluntarily accepts any of the available vaccines is committing mortal sin, because they are condoning and supporting the murder of unborn babies. But that is not the only reason why taking the vaccine is a sin.

The body is a gift from God. ("Know ye not that your bodies are the members of Christ?" 1 Corinthians 6:15) Therefore, harming the body in any way is sinful and the more damage one does to their body, the greater the sin.

Take suicide. We all know that suicide is a mortal sin. Anyone who commits suicide goes straight to hell where they burn in fire and are tortured by demons for all eternity. No one disputes that.

Intentionally harming the body through drug abuse or drunkenness is also a mortal sin. Does that surprise you? It shouldn't. The Bible is very clear on the subject.

St. Paul specifically singles out drunkenness as a mortal sin in Galatians 5:21 when he writes: "Envyings, murders, drunkenness, revellings, and such like: of the which I tell you before, as I have also told you in time past, that they which do such things shall not inherit the kingdom of God."

As you can see in the passage above, St. Paul puts drunkenness on a par with murder as far as its seriousness as a sin. Both are sufficient to condemn one's soul to hell. You may not agree with that, but that's what he says.

A year later, St. Paul wrote in 1 Corinthians 6:10: "Nor thieves, nor covetous nor drunkards, nor revilers, nor extortioners, shall inherit the kingdom of God."

There it is again. St. Paul insisting that those who engage in drunkenness will not inherit the kingdom of God. In other words, they go to hell. In other words, drunkenness is a mortal sin.

And if the act of getting drunk is a mortal sin, how much more of a sin is it to ingest something infinitely more harmful than alcohol, something that can cause permanent damage or even death like the current vaccines?

Deaths and Side Effects

As of this writing, August 2021, over 100,000 people worldwide have died after taking the COVID-19 vaccine. Millions more have suffered serious side effects ranging from permanent paralysis to strokes to blood clotting to heart disease. Those aren't exaggerated numbers either, if anything they're conservative.

The Center for Disease Control's own reporting system, VAERS, says the vaccine has led to over 500,000 deaths, serious injuries and side effects in the United States alone. That's more deaths and injuries than have been caused by every other vaccine over the last thirty years combined.

What's more, the vast majority (over 70%) of those currently testing positive for the alleged virus and its "delta variants," along with over 50% of those whose deaths are attributed to the alleged virus are people who have already been vaccinated, which means the jab really offers no protection at all from the virus. Why do you think everyone that is already fully vaccinated is now being pressured to take a booster shot? Why do you think we are now being told that the shots will have to be annual for life?

A website in the U.K.—www.dailyexpose.co.uk—has an article that claims medical regulators in both the U.S. and U.K. knew in October of 2020 that the injections would cause blood-clots, heart disease, paralysis, harm to children, and even deaths, but they ignored all of that and went ahead pushing the untested vaccines anyway. These are the type of people you're dealing with.

By the way, they're not taking their own vaccines. The heads of all of the vaccine companies are refusing to take their own medicine, and at least one of them is on record saying he's not taking the jab because he's healthy and not at risk. But they demand you take it.

100,000 Deaths or a Six-Pack of Beer?

Now that you know how harmful these untested vaccines actually are, can you see how willfully injecting any of them is a mortal sin?

Can you see how much more damaging a single one of these shots is compared to someone who drinks a six-pack of beer and ends up drunk?

Can you also see how claiming you were coerced into taking the vaccine by the threat of losing your job is a sin?

But it's your job, you cry! There are other jobs and other ways of making a living. To commit mortal sin for the convenience of a cushy job is as lame of an excuse as any person can think of. Would you rather dust off your resume and find something else, or commit mortal sin and risk burning in the fires of hell?

In the United States, companies and institutions have been outright criminal in trying to force their employees and customers to submit to the jab. The NFL has been particularly nasty in trying to force compliance, firing coaches and enacting extremely harsh penalties on the few remaining players with the good sense to just say no.

As I type these words, recently vaxxed Vinny Curry, defensive end for the New York Jets, has just been hospitalized with blood clots. He had to have his spleen removed and is done for the season before it even started. He'll likely never play sports again. And you still want to watch football?

I suspect that all of the companies and institutions pushing mandatory vaccinations on their employees and customers are receiving massive financial kickbacks. Why else would they be doing it?

The people that run these companies and institutions aren't complete ignoramuses—well, some of them aren't. And we know that none of this has anything to do with public health. The only logical explanation for their behavior is they are receiving financial kickbacks of such magnitude that it overshadows the financial losses of their actions. Think about that one.

Now if you're forcibly held down while someone injects you that is not a sin. That scenario is no different than if you were held down while someone forced open your mouth and poured a quart of whisky down your throat; or if someone slipped a narcotic into your drink without you knowing it. None of those would be a sin on your part.

Forced vaccination like that is the endgame, by the way. It's what's planned for humanity by the Satanists running the show, but we're not there yet.

What About the Ignorant?

I suppose one could claim ignorance; could claim that they didn't know taking the jab was a sin. But I doubt if that excuse will fly with God.

Ignorance is a sin in and of itself. Anyone over the age of reason, generally considered to be around 12-years-old, is expected to know the difference between right and wrong and they are expected to act accordingly. So ignorance is no excuse.

Ignorance is a form of dishonesty. It exists only because people are too lazy, too indifferent, or too stupid to seek the truth. That's not meant to berate you if you've already taken the jab. We're all ignorant at one time or another.

Thanks to our media and our modern education system, I was ignorant about history, politics, society, racial differences, religion, the nature of evil in the world and many other things for the first twenty-five years of my life. And I'm still sifting through the lies.

By the way, everything we've covered thus far applies in spades to anyone involved in administering the jab on any level. Whether they actually injected someone or spent any time at all promoting it, they are guilty of serious sin.

That includes politicians and government officials, employers and managers, school officials and teachers, journalists and reporters, bloggers and social media posters, even friends and family members who urged others to take the jab.

Such individuals are in a state of mortal sin. They need to cease sinning immediately and confess what they have already done to a validly ordained priest in order to have any chance at all of escaping eternal damnation.

The Innocence of Children

And the worst of the worst, the biggest mortal sinners of all, are those responsible for promoting or administering the jab to children.

Politicians, health officials, doctors, nurses, teachers, school officials, and parents fall into this class in droves.

They are guilty of one the worst sins imaginable: harming children.

As Jesus said in Luke 17:2: "It were better for him that a millstone were hanged about his neck and he cast into the sea, than that he should offend one of these little ones."

Barring repentance and confession to a validly ordained priest, anyone involved on any level with administering the jab to children is going to burn in hell for all eternity.

I shudder to think of the fate that awaits them.

Pray for Forgiveness

So what if you're one of those guilty parties? What if you've already taken the jab? Or worse, what if you administered the jab to someone else or promoted it in any way? What then?

I would advise you to say an immediate Act of Contrition. By immediate, I mean right now, this very instant as you're reading this. Recite an immediate Act of Contrition and then pray for forgiveness and confess your sin as quickly as possible to a validly ordained priest (a priest ordained before 1968).

Then do whatever you can to reverse the damage done by the vaccine. (Read *Reversing the Side Effects of the COVID-19 Vaccine: How to Heal Yourself of Adverse Reactions to the Vaccine and Protect Yourself from Shedding*.)

Pray and ask forgiveness, not just for this sin, but also for other sins you have committed. If you're not already a traditional Catholic, you must become one immediately. The key word in that last sentence is *traditional.*

To be a traditional Catholic is to reject the changes that came with Vatican II, including the non-Catholic and invalid New Mass, and to completely reject the long line of heretical anti-popes that have occupied the Vatican since the late 1950s.

That list of anti-popes includes John XXIII, John VI, John Paul II, Benedict XVI and Francis.

Those men are all heretical anti-popes. Yes, even John Paul II. In fact, he might be the most heretical of all. Here's a partial list of the sins that "Saint" John Paul II engaged in:

John Paul II taught that those outside the Catholic Church can be saved.

John Paul II taught that non-Christian religions, such as Wicca (Witchcraft) and Satanism were inspired by the Holy Ghost.

John Paul II taught the every man is God: "You are the Christ, the Son of the Living God." The Bible says this is one of the signs of the antichrist.

John Paul II referred to Buddha as "Lord Buddha" and bowed before a statue of Buddha in a Buddhist temple.

John Paul II organized a World Day of Prayer for Peace attended by the leaders of dozens of false religions.

John Paul II approved the use of altar girls.

John Paul II invited Satanists to pray at the Vatican and removed or covered all crucifixes so they would not be seen.

John Paul II prayed with Satanists and participated in voodoo ceremonies.

John Paul II kissed the Koran.

John Paul II spoke at a Lutheran temple.

John Paul II participated in Anglican services.

John Paul II taught that Christians and Muslims worship the same God.

John Paul II allowed himself to be "blessed' by an Indian Shaman.

John Paul II attempted to alter the Rosary!

John Paul II carried the "Broken Cross", a symbol of Satanism.

Bear in mind that Catholic dogma tells us that any one of these aforementioned sins by itself is sufficient to separate one from the Church and condemn their soul to hell. John Paul II was guilty of all of them, plus a whole lot more. This is only a partial list.

The Catholic Encyclopedia of 1914 explains the situation very succinctly: "The pope himself, if notoriously guilty of heresy, would cease to be pope because he would cease to be a member of the Church."

Get it? Anyone, even a person who claims to be Pope, who commits heresy, ceases to be Catholic.

For more on the subject of traditional Catholicism, visit the website www.VaticanCatholic.com and read the book *The*

Truth about What Really Happened to the Catholic Church after Vatican II by Brother Michael Dimond and Brother Peter Dimond. That book is where I found this partial list of John Paul II's heresies.

Seriously, without delay, you must research and investigate traditional Catholicism for yourself. Put aside the bigotry of the anti-Catholics who have never researched the issue for themselves. Pay no attention to the pencil-neck geeks who tell you the Catholic Church is evil. They are speaking about the post Vatican II counterfeit church, not the real Catholic Church. In their ignorance, they don't know the difference.

Use the brain that God gave you and research the issue for yourself. Your eternal salvation depends on it.

How to Say an Act of Contrition

The Act of Contrition is a prayer that one uses to seek forgiveness from God. It should be said immediately after any sin a person commits.

Shortly before World War II began, soldiers and civilians throughout Germany, Poland, France, Italy, Spain, and all of Christian Europe were advised to say an Act of Contrition as a means of receiving forgiveness in the coming war when priests would be scarce and often not available. Soldiers on the battlefield were often forced to recite the Act of

Contrition as their only means of seeking forgiveness. Many souls were likely saved that way.

One priest wrote the following:

"Whoever can, should receive the Sacrament of Penance. Whoever cannot, because of prohibiting circumstances, should cleanse his soul by acts of perfect contrition; i.e, the sorrow of a loving child who does not consider so much the pain or reward as he does the pardon from his father and mother to whom he has brought displeasure."

Here's how to say an Act of Contrition:

Act of Contrition

O my God, I am heartily sorry for having offended Thee,
and I detest all my sins, because I dread the loss of Heaven
and the pains of hell, but most of all because they offend
Thee, my God, Who are all good and deserving of all my love.
I firmly resolve, with the help of Thy grace, to confess my
sins, to do penance, and to amend my life. Amen.

Chapter Four

Is Wearing a Face Mask a Sin?

We've established that taking the COVID-19 vaccine is a serious sin, and an even greater sin for those promoting and administering it, especially to children. But what about wearing a mask?

Is that a sin too?

Actually, it is.

Every child knows that telling a lie is a sin. Donning a face mask under the guise of a fake pandemic is a form of lying.

The mask-wearer didn't concoct the lie himself, but he is giving truth to the lie and doing so in a public manner which influences others to believe it. Thus he is helping to spread a lie.

To better understand this, consider a movie or theatrical play. You have actors playing leading parts and you have actors playing extras. Both have a duty to suspend the disbelief of the viewing public. Both are responsible for the success of the production.

The mask-wearer is an extra on the stage of life. He is not playing a major role, but his participation is necessary for the success of the production. Without his unwitting cooperation, the show would not succeed.

In other words, if the mindless zombies that populate America would just remove their face diapers, the entire hoax would crumble and cease to exist.

Did that last sentence make you cringe?

Did it just send your blood pressure skyrocketing?

Did it jangle the bones of your skull with detonations of cognitive dissonance?

If so, congratulations.

You've taken the first step in educating yourself and possibly saving your soul. Because at this point it's obvious to anyone with a brain in their head that virus mania is nothing more than a charade, a farce, a massive hoax. Anyone who denies that is simply not living in reality.

By hoax, I mean exactly that. No virus, no pandemic, no one dying from an alleged virus, no nothing.

Did you know that a coronavirus is nothing more than a common cold virus? You can research that yourself in any virology textbook.

Did you know that what we're told is the COVID-19 virus has never been isolated, thus it does not even exist? In a recent Canadian court case that you likely never heard of,

Patrick King, a private citizen in Alberta, Canada represented himself in court after being fined $1,200 for protesting the hoax. King subpoenaed the Provincial Health Minister, Dr. Deena Hinshaw, for proof that the COVID-19 virus actually exists.

Guess what happened?

The Health Minister was forced to admit in court that they have no evidence that the virus actually exists because it has never been isolated!

Since that landmark court case took place, the Province has rescinded all COVID restrictions, because they don't have the legal standing to enforce them over a nonexistent virus.

Did you know that not one person in the entire world has actually died from what we are told is the COVID-19 virus? People have died from cancer and heart attacks and car accidents and from falling off ladders and their deaths have been *attributed* to COVID-19, but not one person has actually died from it. How could they when it doesn't exist?

Welcome to the Rabbit Hole.

Exploding Heads

At this precise point, roughly half of the people reading this book are experiencing massive reality shock. Some are sputtering and foaming at the mouth. Others are hurling the book across the room. A few wise ones are stroking their chin and saying, "This is interesting ..."

If it's hard for you to wrap your head around the entire pandemic being nothing more than a hoax, you're not alone. Many good men and good women experienced the exact same thing when they first learned that 9/11 was an inside job, or that Lee Harvey Oswald never fired a shot at John F. Kennedy.

Society has become so fake that the truth actually hurts people. They find it so startling, so alien to the brainwashing they've been subjected to that they simply can't believe it's real no matter how much evidence you show them.

A normal person's first reaction to truthful information is anger, followed by denial, and then–if they actually take the time to research the issue–acceptance of the truth. You may have to go through the exact same phases as part of your growth process.

I remember when I first heard that global warming was a fraud. I was so brainwashed by school and by the media at the time that I thought the idea was preposterous. But I researched it, if only to prove the charge was false. And lo and behold, what did I find? I found that global warming *was* a fraud. A complete and total fraud. What an eye-opener that was.

The question now is or you man enough or woman enough to handle the truth? Most people aren't. Most people prefer to have others do their thinking for them. They cower like frightened chickens when confronted with the truth and do everything they can to avoid knowing it.

Patrick King of Canada has given us all an inspiring demonstration of the power of one person, and what a single courageous citizen can accomplish.

How about you?

The "Tell" of the Century

When someone is bluffing in poker, they often exhibit what's known as a "tell." A "tell" is something that gives them away, a mannerism, an action, a spoken word or inflection of voice, some kind of signal that exposes the lie. Liars do this in real life, as well, and a trained eye can easily spot it.

Do you remember back in the spring and summer of 2020 how the big, bad virus miraculously disappeared every time a "mostly peaceful protest" erupted?

Do you remember how all of those dancing nurses and heroic "health care" workers–the ones who called mask and lockdown protesters "criminals" and accused them of murder–suddenly flipped and said it was perfectly fine for tens of thousands of violent criminals to riot, loot and burn down businesses without wearing masks and without social distancing?

Do you remember how not one of those violent rioters or their idiot followers ever came down with the "virus"?

I remember that. If the behavior of everyone involved is not a "tell," I don't know what is.

Truth or Lie

There is no escaping the truth. A person is either telling the truth or they are lying. You can't do both at the same time. And if someone is lying, they are committing a sin and at risk of eternal damnation.

Each of us has an obligation, a duty, to learn the truth and to expose falsehoods and lies. Those who turn their back on reality, who turn their nose up at facts and ignore truthful evidence, because reality, facts and evidence make them uncomfortable, are not just harming themselves, they are also harming everyone they come in contact with. Thus, their actions are contributing to the sins of others and putting their own soul in even deeper jeopardy that it already is. They're also contributing to the continual dumbing-down and general stupidity of society.

Dishonesty in any form is a sin. When one chooses to wear a mask they are participating in dishonesty by giving truth to a lie. Thus, they are committing a sin.

Even for Five Minutes?

If the grocery store won't let you in without a mask and you need to buy food in order to survive, then donning a mask for five minutes while you gather your groceries is not a sin. To allow yourself or your family to starve would be a greater sin than wearing a mask for five minutes.

If your brainwashed boss insists you wear a mask in order to keep your job, then it's not a sin for you to do so. Depriving yourself and your family of a means of support would be a greater sin. Hopefully, you can find another job, working for somebody with an ounce of intelligence.

What is a sin is to voluntarily wear a mask for anything that's not essential to your survival. In your heart, you know what that means.

Wearing a mask in order to board a plane to go on vacation or to go to Disneyland or to Las Vegas is a sin. (Going to either of those places with or without a mask is a sin.)

Wearing a mask to go shopping at the mall or to any non-essential store is a sin.

Wearing a mask to attend a movie, concert or sporting event is a sin. (After the three major sports leagues–football, baseball, and basketball–all came out in support of sodomy, rioting, looting, violence, cities being burned to the ground and more last year, anyone with a desire to attend any type of professional sporting event ever again needs to have their head examined.)

Wearing a mask to enter a nightclub or bar is a sin.

Wearing a mask while you walk down the sidewalk, walk your dog, or water your lawn is a sin.

I think you get the idea. It's a matter of whether the activity that's demanding that you wear a mask is essential to your survival or not. Shopping for food is essential. Shopping for clothes, cosmetics, furniture, electronics and other nonsense is not.

Wearing a mask merely for convenience is a sin.

Wearing a mask in order to fit in with the crowd–one of the primary reasons why everyone is doing it–is a sin.

Wearing a mask in your social media avatar is not only a sin it's no different than wearing a sign around your neck that says: I AM AN IDIOT.

A Coward Dies a Thousand Deaths

Wearing a mask is also a sign of cowardice. God didn't create you to grovel, to don a submission diaper and crawl on your knees like a slave. He created you to stand tall as a man, or as a woman; to face life courageously and with faith. How hurt and insulted God must be to see his beautiful creations voluntarily silencing themselves with face masks and crawling in the dirt like worms.

They say crisis reveals character. Nowhere has that been more evident than over the last two years. Feminized men hiding behind face diapers, bawling like babies for others to do the same. Witless women doing exactly the same thing. Absolutely disgusting.

Remember those phony videos from China we saw back in February of 2020 with people collapsing in the street and dying from the big, bad virus? People saw those videos, panicked, and then stampeded the supermarket where they created scenes of mass hysteria, overloaded their shopping carts, and fought each other for toilet paper. Remember?

Those scenes of supermarket chaos and hoarding were conveniently captured on film and then broadcast to the world, which only created more fear and more panic among the populace.

Now here we are, a full year and a half later and nobody has collapsed in the street, nobody has died from the alleged virus, and nobody knows anyone that has died from it, yet everyone knows multiple people that have died or are suffering serious side effects from the vaccine.

Crazy, isn't it? And none of it would be happening without a multitude of frightened sheep giving it power by wearing their face diapers.

Lying is Bad for Your Health

Lying is not only a sin, it's also crippling to our health. Every time we lie, every time we perform a dishonest act, every time we give truth to a lie in any way (such as agreeing with a lie, giving public support to a lie, or refusing to expose a lie, which we do every time we put on a face mask), we weaken our immune system.

You can prove this to yourself quite easily with simple kinesiology. Kinesiology is a form of muscle testing that acts as an instant lie detector. Unlike the polygraph tests administered by law enforcement, kinesiology is 100% accurate. It can also be used to determine whether a product, person or place is beneficial to you or not.

Make a truthful statement while using kinesiology to test your muscle's ability to resist and you'll see that your body's response is strong. Then test the same muscle while making a false statement and watch how weak the body becomes.

Now imagine the damage that's being done to a person's immune system when they choose to live a dishonest life, week by week, day by day, hour by hour. It's happening all around us.

One of the worst lies of all is the adult to child lie. There's the child, wide-eyed and innocent and looking for answers from the adult they trust. And then there's the adult, usually a parent or teacher, regurgitating some ridiculous lie they just saw on television.

Granted, some of those parents and teachers are ignorant of the lies they spew. They actually believe what they see on the boob tube. Many of them are so gullible they believe the virus hoax. But, as we said earlier, ignorance is not an excuse.

To seek Heaven on one hand, while clinging to a life of lies on the other, makes your chances of success very slim. It's important to come clean, to admit when you've been fooled, and embrace the truth.

There's no shame in admitting you're been conned. When I was in grade school, high school and college, I believed every word of nonsense my parents and my teachers told me. Looking back, it was a non-stop litany of lies, some of it well-intentioned, but almost all of it brimming with dishonesty.

But I bought it. I bought all of it. It was a mistake and today I admit it. There's no harm in doing the same if you've been conned by the virus hoax.

Refusal to admit a mistake stems from pride. Pride is one of the seven capital sins, along with covetousness, lust, anger, gluttony, envy and sloth.

Some say pride is the greatest of all sins, because it expresses self-love and is directly opposed to submission to God. As such, they say it is the sin most hated by God and the one He punishes most severely.

Anyone who falls for the virus hoax and refuses to admit it is guilty of the sin of pride.

Follow the Advice of Jacinta from Fatima

Anyone who wants to see Heaven should begin living a totally truthful life. *Totally* truthful, you ask? Yes, totally truthful.

The easiest way to do that is to follow the advice given by little Jacinta of Fatima when she said, "Always tell the truth, even when it is hard."

(Jacinta was one of three seers at Fatima, where the Miracle of the Sun took place. The Miracle of the Sun is one of the greatest miracles in the history of the world, certainly the greatest miracle since the Resurrection. To learn more about Fatima and the Miracle of the Sun, I recommend visiting www.VaticanCatholic.com, and reading the books *Our Lady of Fatima*, *The Crusade of Fatima*, and *The Impostor Sister Lucy*.)

For many people, the most difficult part of living a totally truthful life is admitting that they currently lie. So they won't do it. Instead, they'll continue to lie by claiming they live an honest life.

Charging too much for a product, service, housing or rent is a form of lying.

People who are guilty of such a lie will immediately draw themselves up and claim that such a statement is not true. They'll say they are merely charging "what they are worth" or charging "fair market value." But that is just another lie.

False or misleading advertising is a form of lying.

Teaching fake history in a classroom is a form of lying.

Pushing drugs, unnecessary surgery, or radiation treatments and calling yourself a doctor is a form of lying.

Donning a face mask under the guise of a fake pandemic is a form of lying.

Tell the Truth and Look Instantly Younger

Those with a touch of vanity, and I confess to having a little myself, will be happy to hear that a side effect from living a totally truthful life is you begin to look younger.

It takes a lot of energy and stress to hold back the truth. Once you release that energy and allow the truth to flow easily through your body, your facial features soften and the years melt away like a snow cone on a hot summer day. It's really quite amazing and you will notice it on yourself if you begin living a totally truthful life.

Of course, the flip side to that are those who live their entire life under a cloak of lies. Look at the people pushing the virus hoax the hardest:

Bill Gates is 65 and looks 80. His face is lined and creased with age far beyond his years.

Recently disgraced Anthony Cuomo looks 15 to 20 years older than his age.

Anthony Fauci looks like a wrinkled old dwarf.

Klaus Schwab has been bald almost his entire life and looks like he has one foot in the grave.

George Soros looks like death warmed over.

Look at others known for twisting the truth:

Bill Clinton, a handsome man during his presidency, has deteriorated rapidly.

Barack Obama's hair has turned gray overnight and his face has aged considerably. He looks like a wrinkled old prune.

Hillary looks like the Goodyear Blimp.

And on and on.

The good news for these folks and others is that any one of them could immediately knock years off their appearance and begin to look and feel much younger if they would just stop lying.

The bad news is none of them are likely to do that.

Chapter Five

Is COVID-19 the Mark of the Beast?

The final book of the Bible is called Revelations or The Apocalypse. It contains prophecies of the tribulations the Church will face in the last days, as well as various events that will transpire at the end of the world.

Some say the last days are yet to come, but they are mistaken. The last days are not some future event yet to come. They are happening right now. We're living through them.

You can prove to this to yourself quite easily by studying the prophecies from Revelations that have come true over the last several decades. The Dimond brothers at Most Holy Family Monastery have performed excellent research in this regard. Let's look at a couple of things they've discovered, beginning with Revelations 12:1.

The Douay-Rheims Bible says: "And a great sign appeared in heaven: A woman clothed with the sun, and the moon under her feet, and on her head a crown of twelve stars."

That prophecy was fulfilled on October 13, 1917 when the sun danced in the sky before 70,000 eyewitnesses at Fatima, Portugal. It's known as the Miracle of the Sun and it is one of the greatest miracles in the history of the world.

The Bible's exact words are: "A woman clothed with the sun, and the moon under her feet ..." That is exactly how the Virgin Mary appears in her supernatural imprint on the cloak of Juan Diego from Guadalupe, Mexico–another great miracle; a miracle that put an end to the practice of human sacrifice among the Aztec Indians and resulted in the conversion of over eight million Indians from paganism to Christianity, thus saving their souls.

The words "clothed with the sun" also describe to a "T" the Miracle of the Sun at Fatima, which took place at the final apparition of the Virgin Mary to three local children.

The local Masonic newspaper, *O Seculo*, sent their editor to the event to ridicule it, but even he came away a believer. The paper's headline in describing the event read: Astounding Things! How the Midday Sun Danced at Fatima; The Apparitions of the Virgin–What the Sign from Heaven Consisted of–Many Thousands of People Confirm a Miracle Occurred–War and Peace.

Notice how the paper's headline inadvertently confirmed the fulfillment of the prophecy by using almost the exact same words as the Bible.

The Bible says: "a great sign appeared in Heaven," and then describes the Virgin Mary.

O Seculo credits the Virgin Mary for the miracle by saying: "The Apparitions of the Virgin" and then adds: "What the Sign from Heaven Consisted of."

And that from a Masonic newspaper.

You may not know this, but when a Freemason reaches the 33rd degree, they are entrusted with a great secret: Masons worship Lucifer. So for a Masonic newspaper, dedicated to Satanism, to confirm Biblical prophecy is the ultimate jiu-jitsu move by God. It's presenting evidence of the fulfillment of this prophecy that even the most willfully blind person cannot fail to see.

That we are currently living in the end times was further confirmed by Sister Lucy, one of the three seers of Fatima. In her last public interview on December 26, 1957 with Father Fuentes, she said, "Father, the Most Holy Virgin did not tell me that we are in the last times of the world, but she made me understand this for three reasons.

"The first reason is because she told me that the devil is about to engage in a decisive battle with the Holy Virgin, and a decisive battle is a final battle where one side will be victorious and the other side will suffer defeat. Hence from now on we are for God or we are for the devil. There is no middle course.

"The second reason is because she said to my cousins as well as to myself that God is giving two last remedies to the world: the Holy Rosary and the Devotion to the Immaculate Heart of Mary. These being the last two remedies, this signifies that there will be no others.

"The third reason is because as always in the plans of Divine Providence, God, before He is about to chastise the world, exhausts all other remedies. Now, when He sees that the world pays no attention whatsoever, then, as we say in our imperfect manner of speaking, He offers us with a certain trepidation the last means of salvation, His Most Holy Mother. It is with a certain trepidation because if you despise and repulse this ultimate means we will not have any more forgiveness from Heaven because we will have committed a sin which the Gospel calls the sin against the Holy Ghost. This sin consists of openly rejecting, with full knowledge and consent, the salvation which He offers.

"Remember that Jesus Christ is a very good Son and that He does not permit that we offend and despise His Most Holy Mother. We have as testimony many centuries of Church history which demonstrate, by the terrible chastisements which have befallen those who have attacked the honor of His Most Holy Mother, how Our Lord Jesus Christ has always defended the honor of his Mother.

"Regarding the Holy Rosary, look, Father, the Most Holy Virgin, in these last times in which we live, has given a new efficacy to the recitation of the Rosary. So much so, that there is no problem, no matter how difficult it is, whether temporal or, above all, spiritual, in the personal life of each one of us, of our families, of the families of the world, or of the religious communities, or even of the life of peoples and nations, that cannot be solved by the Rosary.

"There is no problem, I tell you, no matter how difficult it is, that we cannot resolve by praying the Holy Rosary. With the Holy Rosary, we will save ourselves, we will sanctify ourselves, we will console Our Lord and obtain the salvation of many souls."

More Evidence

Here's some more great evidence of Biblical prophecy fulfilled that the Dimond brothers have uncovered:

Revelations 18:2 states: "And he cried mightily with a strong voice, saying: Babylon the great is fallen, is fallen, and is become the habitation of devils and the hold of every foul spirit, and a cage of every unclean and hateful bird."

The beginning of the verse, the part that states: "And he cried mightily with a strong voice, saying Babylon the great is fallen, is fallen", was fulfilled on February 12, 2013 when St. Peter's Basilica was struck twice by lightning.

Babylon refers to Rome. We know this because St. Peter wrote his first epistle while he was in Rome and in that epistle he refers to Rome as Babylon: "The church that is at Babylon, elected together with you, saluteth you ..." 1 St. Peter 5:13.

The word "fallen" refers to Jesus' words in Luke 10:18: "And he said unto them: I beheld Satan as lightning fall from heaven."

So when St. John writes in Revelations: "Babylon the great is fallen, is fallen," he is prophesizing how the once great city of Rome where the Vatican is located will fall to Satan. That did indeed happen with the advent of Vatican II in the 1960s.

Notice how the words "is fallen," which reference Satan falling like lightning from heaven, are repeated twice. We then see a visible sign from heaven that this prophecy has been fulfilled by lightning twice striking St. Peter's Basilica.

The Habitation of Devils

The second part of Revelations 18:2 which states: "and is become the habitation of devils and the hold of every foul spirit, and a cage of every unclean and hateful bird" was fulfilled on December 8, 2015 when anti-pope Francis put on a light show at the Vatican.

At this light show, images of birds, snakes, reptiles, and other animals, as well as Buddhist "monks" and devilish faces were projected onto the twelve pillars in front of St. Peter's Basilica.

You can view this demonic light show for yourself, although I wouldn't recommend it. If you do watch it, picture yourself as St. John back in the first century A.D., before television, before video, before sound recording, before any of the technology we now possess and imagine how he would have described such an event, along with lightning twice striking St. Peter's Basilica. The answer is exactly how he did describe it in Revelations 18:2: "Babylon the great is fallen, is fallen: and is become the habitation of devils and the hold of every foul spirit, and a cage of every unclean and hateful bird."

Note that when St. John saw this vision of Babylon (Rome, home of the Catholic Church) as "a cage of every unclean and hateful bird," he saw it exactly as the spectators of anti-pope Francis' light show did. The projection of birds and other creatures against St. Peter's Basilica looked precisely like caged creatures, with the twelve pillars of the Basilica appearing to be the bars of a cage.

Here again, we see evidence so crystal clear that this prophecy has been fulfilled in our time that only the most dense and muddle-brained individual can fail to grasp it.

The Mark of the Beast

Now let's look at perhaps the most famous lines in all of Revelations. Here I'm going to present my own thoughts, not those of the Dimond brothers. Revelations 13:16-18 states: "And he causeth all, both small and great, rich and poor, free and bond, to receive a mark in their right hand, or in their character in their foreheads:

"And that no man might buy or sell, save he that had the mark, or the name of the beast, or the number of his name.

"Here is wisdom. Let him that hath understanding, count the number of the beast: for it is the number of a man; and his number is six hundred threescore and six."

Does that sound like anything we're going through now?

As I type these words, France has mandated a country-wide vaccine passport. Without proof of vaccination, no one is allowed inside any business or building, including supermarkets. In other words, it's required to buy or sell. Without it, you cannot buy food. Without it, you will starve to death.

The mayor of Lapu-Lapu in the Philippines is not allowing anyone who is unvaccinated to buy food or groceries.

Australia is close behind. They are currently experiencing draconian lockdowns and will likely initiate their own vaccine passport very soon. There's plenty of talk about doing the same in the United States with initial trials currently underway in New York, San Francisco and Los Angeles.

Is this all just a giant coincidence?

Before you answer, consider this verse from Revelations 18:23: "For thy merchants were the great men of the earth; for by thy sorceries were all nations deceived."

Look up the word *sorceries* in *Strong's Concordance*, a reference book that lists the Hebrew and Greek translation of every word in the Bible, and you'll find that the original Greek meaning for sorceries is pharmakeia or pharmacy. In other words, the Bible considers pharmaceutical drug medications to be sorcery and witchcraft.

Therefore, what that line of prophecy is really saying is: "For thy merchants were the great men of the earth: for by thy drug medications were all nations deceived."

Sound familiar?

Or is this another coincidence?

But wait, there's more.

House of Representatives Bill 6666

Have you heard of H.R. Bill 6666? Introduced by U.S. Representative Bobby Rush and supported by 58 Democrats and 1 Republican co-sponsor, it proposes the most massive spy program on American citizens ever, all under the guise of COVID-19.

Among the bill's draconian language is this: "trace and monitor the contacts of infected individuals and to support the quarantine of such individuals through mobile health units."

Know what that means? It means if you politely refuse to be jabbed or if you receive a false positive test for the imaginary virus—and the testing protocol is riddled with false positives—you can be hauled away in a "mobile health unit" to an internment camp and locked up for life. No trial, no due process, no nothing. Sound like fun?

Do you think it's a coincidence that the bill is numbered 6666?

But wait, we're still not finished.

Depopulation by Vaccine

Remember Bill Gates? He's the guy who in 2010 said, "The world today has 6.8 billion people. That's headed up to about 9 billion. Now, if we do a really great job on new vaccines, health care, reproductive health services, we could lower that by perhaps 10 or 15 percent."

That's an exact quote. You can look it up. Watch how excited Gates gets when he talks about lowering the human population through vaccines and then ask yourself just who is getting these vaccines?

The answer, of course, is live people.

So to lower the human population by means of vaccines can have only two meanings: sterilization or death.

In 2019, Gates filed a patent application entitled *Crypto Currency System Using Human Body Activity Data.*

It's exactly what it says it is; a crypto currency system designed to eliminate cash. And just how will this "human body activity data" be transmitted and processed in order to buy and sell? By an embedded microchip, of course.

Can you guess what this patent application number is? It's WO/2020/060606.

Do you think that patent number with its triple sixes is a coincidence?

Remember, this is the same Bill Gates whose manly wife wears an upside cross, a symbol of Satanism.

This is the same Bill Gates whose company partnered with "spirit cooking" artist Marina Abramovic, an alleged Satanist, and released a commercial starring her on Good Friday. And this is the same Marina Abramovic who proudly posed with Jacob Rothschild before a painting titled *Satan Summoning His Legions*.

But I guess those are all just coincidences too.

Klaus Schwab

Are you familiar with Klaus Schwab? He is the founder and chairman of the World Economic Forum in Davos, Switzerland, which annually brings together the heads of state of the world's major countries to discuss the future of world affairs. In other words, Schwab is a major player on the world stage and one of the most influential men on earth. When he says, "Jump," presidents of major countries say, "How high?"

In an interview with Swiss channel RTS on January 10, 2016, a full four years before our current "pandemic," Schwab explained how every human being on earth will soon be micro-chipped in order to merge with the digital world.

Schwab, in glowing terms, described how microchips imbedded in the skin or in the brain of all humans is inevitable and that these microchips will be necessary for people in order to buy or sell.

The interviewer asked Schwab when this would take place, and Schwab responded, "Certainly in the next ten years." That was five years ago, which puts us on track for a micro-chipped population right now.

Some say the COVID-19 RNA (mRNA) injections are designed to reprogram people's DNA by removing the God gene and turning them into walking, talking genetically modified organisms. As such, they are no longer considered human in the legal sense, but rather the property of those who injected them and those who own the vaccine patents.

If the herd of humanity continues to submit to these injections, we're looking at a world in which everyone will have to be micro-chipped and connected to the "system" via 5G technology in order to do anything. If you refuse, the system will refuse you. You won't be able to buy or sell. You won't be able to eat.

Schwab and others like him envision a future in which natural humans with God-implanted DNA no longer exist, replaced by a population of micro-chipped transhumanist creatures. This is their future and they can't wait for it to happen.

They want to replace God's creations with their own creations. In essence, they want to become gods themselves. Someone else tried that once. Do you remember who it was?

Another Coincidence?

Tell me if this is a coincidence.

Number the letters of the alphabet, beginning with the number 1 for A, the number 2 for B, etc., up to the number 26 for Z.

Next take the word CORONA and assign the proper number from your list to each letter. For instance, the letter C is 3, the letter O is 15, the letter R is 18 etc.

When you are finished, add the numbers up. The result is 66.

Now count the number of letters in the word CORONA. The answer is 6.

Add that number 6 to the numerical coding of the word CORONA which we've already determined is 66 and the result is 666.

"Let him that hath understanding, count the number of the beast: for it is the number of a man; and his number is six hundred threescore and six."

A	B	C	D	E	F	G	H	I
1	2	3	4	5	6	7	8	9
J	K	L	M	N	O	P	Q	R
10	11	12	13	14	15	16	17	18
S	T	U	V	W	X	Y	Z	
19	20	21	22	23	24	25	26	

CORONA = 6 letters

C	3
O	15
R	18
O	15
N	14
A	1
6 letters = 6	66

Like everything else we've discussed, it's possible that this is merely another coincidence. Coincidence number 666.

It's also possible that U.S. Representative Bobby Rush requested bill number 6666 as a joke or to troll people.

And it's possible that Bill Gates did the same thing with his patent number WO/2020/060606. He may have meant it as a joke too. But why would he do that?

Why would anyone who supposedly cares for people and wants to help them and who has humanity's best interests at heart deliberately frighten and insult millions of Christians by doing such a thing?

Why would Bobby Rush do it?

Why does Klaus Schwab want to microchip all of us?

Why is Schwab so insistent that humans be forcibly injected against their will?

Why does Schwab want to transform us all from living, breathing human beings into transhumanist creations?

Why does Schwab get so excited when he talks of turning us all into cyborgs?

Is COVID-19 the Mark of the Beast?

So we're left with the ultimate question: is COVID-19 with its vaccines and vaccine passports the Mark of the Beast as prophesied in the Bible? The evidence that we've examined and the push to make the vaccine mandatory for everyone on earth in order to buy or sell suggests that it either is the Mark of the Beast, or the frontrunner to it, but neither I nor anyone else can answer that question for sure.

We know that anyone taking the Mark of the Beast will not enter the gates of Heaven. Therefore, if COVID-19 *is* in any way related to this prophecy from Revelations, we cannot accept it under any circumstances. Therefore, the only logical response for anyone who wants to go to Heaven is to not have anything to do with it.

We also know that even if COVID-19 isn't related to the Mark of the Beast, everything about it is cloaked in evil therefore we should still avoid it. Failure to do so puts our soul at risk of eternal damnation.

Those are my thoughts.

The Dimond brothers, Michael and Peter, of Most Holy Family Monastery have a different take on the subject. They are the world's leading experts on Catholic doctrine and Biblical prophecy, so I strongly suggest you research their material at www.VaticanCatholic.com

Anyone, Catholic or not, needs to visit their site.

At this point in time, nothing else matters in the world. This issue is the dividing point between all peoples, between all races and between all political affiliations. You either submit to the jab or you don't.

And for those who don't submit, a sea of tribulations await.

Chapter Six

America

"America where are you now?
"Don't you care about your sons and daughters?"
– Steppenwolf - *Monster/Suicide/America*

The United States of America, the greatest country in the history of the world; the country that has done more good for more people than all of the other countries throughout the entire history of the world combined, is gone.

Finished.

Kaput.

The United States is now a 21st century representation of the ancient Roman Empire. Paganism run amok, anti-Christian, anti-family and anti-life. A society saturated with sexual perversion and dripping with evil, all of it cleverly cloaked in the guise of consumerism. America is dead.

This is a sad truth that must be faced. There are plenty of patriots all across the land who were willing to give their life for what they believed this country stood for. Today, those same patriots may be forced to give their life defending their family from what this country has become.

America is finished and it's not coming back; not now, not ever. The communists in control are not going to give up their power, and Donald Trump is not going to ride to the rescue in 2024. Anyone counting on that is living in a state of delusion. In fact, Trump is largely responsible for creating the mess we're in. The final nail in the coffin happened on his watch.

Ultimately, of course, the fault lies with all of us, collectively, for allowing it to happen. The country's fall was decades in the making and collectively we sat back and watched it take place.

The old-time America of "Mom, hot dogs and apple pie" that many of us were brainwashed into believing was actually on life support for quite some time. It took this virus hoax and the fake election to finally deliver the fatal kill-shot.

When you think about it, how could it have turned out any other way?

The rise of Communist feminism in the 60s and 70s, and with it legalized abortion, no-fault-divorce, the welfare state, sexual perversion of every sort, and unfettered immigration were sins of such magnitude they upset the natural order of God and doomed our country to destruction.

God will not be mocked. As a country, we turned our backs on Him, and now it is as if God has said, "You don't want to live under my rules? Fine, I'll let Satan run things down there on earth. See how you like that."

The situation calls for a tactical retreat.

Who Has the Ability to Survive?

A tactical retreat is a specific military maneuver. It doesn't mean surrender and it doesn't mean to turn tail and run. It means to pull back and regroup; to make an organized withdrawal from combat while maintaining contact with the enemy.

Dating, mating, procreating ... that's all out the window now.

Growing your company, moving up the corporate ladder, achieving fame and success ... nothing could be more pointless.

Going on vacation, following celebrity gossip, attending concerts, sporting events and movies in the belief that the world is going back to "normal" ... have you lost your mind?

Nothing is ever going back to normal. Ever.

What matters now is survival.

Survival of your physical body, yes, but more importantly the survival of your soul. Because that's what they're really after.

If you have children then you really have to be on guard. You're going to have to be almost superhuman in your efforts to save yourself and them.

It goes without saying that you must homeschool them. Failure to do so exposes them to the lies and corruption of the education system and puts their soul at risk of eternal damnation.

People are out to exterminate you. Even worse, they're out to exterminate your children. And even worse than that, they're out to steal both your and your children's souls.

That's the current state of America today, and indeed the rest of the world.

The only thing that matters now—the only thing that's ever mattered—is saving your soul.

Saving your soul first, and then helping as many other people as possible save their own souls.

Nothing. Else. Matters.

A Community of Like-Minded Christians

The commie pukes can have the country. They stole it, they can have it. It won't do them any good when they pass the veil and find themselves burning for eternity in the fire of hell.

They lack the competency to run the country so it will continue to deteriorate. Poverty and homelessness will increase. Crime, looting and lawlessness will increase. Sexual deviancy will increase as they come for your children. Get ready for hell on earth.

Even worse, those participating in these sins will attempt to drag you down with them.

Remember the expression "Misery loves company"? They're all miserable and they want to make you miserable too. They know they're going to hell and they want to take you and as many other people as they can to hell with them.

Don't let them do it.

The electoral path to reclaiming the country no longer exists on the national or the state level, but it does still exist locally. That's where we need to concentrate our forces.

The ideal situation at this time is to find a community of like-minded traditional Catholics and move there; a community with local political leaders who aren't brainwashed or under some kind of Jeffrey-Epstein-type blackmail, and with a sheriff who knows the score and is committed to uphold the Constitution.

Unfortunately, I am not aware of any such community anywhere in the world.

If you know where one exists, please let me know, I'd like to move there.

Perhaps you can form such a community.

Barring that, you can try developing a virtual community with friends across the globe.

Barring that, you'll have to go it alone.

It won't be easy. But no one ever said going to Heaven was a piece of cake.

Chapter Seven

Land of the Duped

Have you ever studied the effect of advertising on the human brain? If so, then you know that one of advertising's core tenets is that belief is a matter of feeling and emotion rather than of reason.

Another principal of advertising is that belief is dependent on desire. We believe what we want to believe.

A third tenet of advertising holds that belief has a social component. People have a need for conformity, especially with those in authority.

When people are told that a mysterious killer virus is coming to take their lives and the lives of everyone around them it triggers a high degree of emotionalism and fear. That emotion overrides their ability to reason and think logically.

It also creates a strong desire within them for the prognosis to be true and people believe what they want to believe.

Third, it fulfills the need most people have to bow down and subjugate themselves to authority. This is compounded by their need to conform. They see everyone else behaving like little sheep and that compels them to do the same.

These psychological truths and patterns of behavior are rooted in the overwhelming desire most people have to remain forever wrapped in the warm cocoon of childhood, to remain as children in a world of adults.

Part of the appeal to this way of life is just how easy it is to be a child. Being a child requires little to no thinking. The child as adult shows up for work and does what they are told or have been trained to do. Meanwhile, every feeling, every desire and every thought they have about the world has been devised, formulated and put into their head by other people. In other words, they are brainwashed.

Every decision they've ever made in their life—how they dress, the kind of car they drive, the work they do, their political affiliations and beliefs, what they look for in a mate, what attracts them sexually, all it—has been created by someone else and implanted into their mind via a coordinated process of education, advertising, social conditioning, and straight-out propaganda.

Many of them have never had a single original thought in their life. Because their beliefs are not their own they lack the vocabulary to adequately express them. Ask them a question and they'll respond by repeating whatever it is they heard on talk radio or from the talking heads on television, regurgitating the exact same words, talking points and phrases, as if these were their own original thoughts.

This way of life can be very comforting. Living as a child reduces or even eliminates the need to think. For most people that is a tremendous relief, because thinking is hard work. I don't just mean the required reading and research that a thinking person must do, but the actual process of thinking itself, of rubbing two brain cells together. It's tough, and most people find it much easier to daydream about being famous, fantasize about sex, or concern themselves with the lives of celebrities.

Some will deny this.

Those who deny it most heavily are the most heavily brainwashed.

How massive and how ingrained is the brainwashing, you ask?

From the time the virus farce began back in February of 2020 and up until they rolled out the vaccines in the summer of 2021, I was the only person-and I mean the *only* person-within a three mile radius of my neighborhood not wearing a mask. It went on that way for well over a year.

At first, the streets were deserted and I enjoyed being the only person visible on formally crowded city sidewalks. But then slowly they appeared ... zombies in face masks.

Thousands of them.

It got to the point where I had to put a note on the inside of my door, something I would see every day just before leaving the house, to remind myself that everyone I was about to see or meet was mentally deranged.

Once the vaccines came out, I began seeing a handful of others not wearing masks. Today in my neighborhood, it's about 90% masked, 10% unmasked, and I assume the unmasked are vaxxed, otherwise why weren't they unmasked before?

On a typical day I pass around two hundred masked people on the street. Multiply that by eighteen months and you're talking over 109,000 people that I've walked past, all wearing masks. Not one of those 109,000 mask-wearers has asked me why I'm not wearing one. Not one has shown the least bit of curiosity. They shuffle past me in silence, their eyes straight ahead in a fluoride stare, looking like mindless drones.

In some cases, they see me coming and literally step off the sidewalk and onto the street where they scurry around the cars parked on the curb in order to avoid me. That's the level of mental derangement in my neighborhood.

They wear masks in their cars here too. Around 70% of the drivers I see are alone in their cars with the windows rolled up and wearing a mask. I feel like flagging them down and asking if they'd like to buy an outdoor seatbelt to wear when they're not driving.

All summer long the streets here have been packed with mask-wearers. I see half-naked girls in their teens and twenties (they're literally everywhere) and they're all wearing one of those stupid masks. I see people dressed for work, some in suits and others in work clothes, all wearing masks. I see children going to and from school; young ones walking with their parents, older ones alone or in groups. They're all wearing masks.

Every business has a sign on the door demanding everyone who enters to wear a mask. Every business has an employee planted somewhere near the door in order to enforce this mask-wearing policy.

I don't consider myself an exceptionally brave person, but when I see the rampant cowardice of the vaxxed and the mask-wearers, the way they cringe with fear over a non-existent virus, I feel like an adult among children.

"Nuclear War?!...There Goes My Career!"

If you're familiar with pop art, you may have seen Mark Vallen's famous silkscreen print featuring a young woman in tears with the dialogue caption: "Nuclear War?!... There Goes My Career!"

It was made during the height of the Cold War as a satirical comment on those whose selfishness prevented them from seeing that they were responsible for the current state of the country and of the world. Nuclear war and the obliteration of all human life was secondary to their career goals.

Substitute the words "Global Genocide" for "Nuclear War" and that piece of art is as timely as ever. The selfish masses of today care nothing about freedom or independence, care nothing about the health and safety of children, care nothing about the ongoing genocide taking place. All they care about is themselves.

That's why the patience and understanding that the unvaxxed have for the vaxxed is wearing thinner and thinner. The former know that without the compliant sheep of the latter, none of the lockdowns and illegal state mandates would be taking place. The latter whine and cry for life to return to "normal," never stopping to consider that everything would return to normal, exactly the way they want it to, if they would merely stop bowing down to the beast.

In the Bible, 2 Thessalonians 10-11 states: "And with all deceivableness of unrighteousness in them that perish; because they received not the love of the truth, that they might be saved. And for this cause God shall send them strong delusion, that they should believe a lie."

Have you ever read anything so spot-on in your life?

Billions of people—yes, billions—of such bad will that God has allowed them to be deceived. They are literally incapable of knowing the truth.

And they are all on their way to hell.

Chapter Eight

Where Do We Go from Here?

We now know that what the world calls a pandemic is nothing more than a massive hoax. We also know that mankind is currently living in the end times, the last days. So where do we go from here? Are you doomed to suffer eternal damnation if you have already taken the jab?

Not if you're still alive. If you're breathing and have not yet passed the veil, you still have a chance to save your soul. After all, if sorcerers who sell their souls to the devil can still be saved through repentance and conversion, then so can you. But you must act swiftly.

Dozens of medical doctors and scientists around the world, all working independently of each other, have said that everyone receiving the jab will be dead within three to five years.

I have no way of knowing whether that is true or not, but these doctors are not familiar with each other. They number in the hundreds and they have all come to the same conclusion based on their own independent research.

I personally know of ten people who have taken the jab. They range in age from early 20s to mid-90s. Six of them appear perfectly fine. Three became ill immediately after receiving the jab, one of them seriously ill. She had to have surgery. One died, and it wasn't the 95-year-old.

One out of ten dying means taking the jab is akin to playing Russian Roulette. Only instead of one live bullet in a chamber of six, you have a one in ten chance of dying.

If that percentage holds up, we're looking at a 10% reduction of the world's population, close to a billion people killed. That just so happens to match the number of dead people referenced by Bill Gates when he said, "The world today has 6.8 billion people. That's headed up to about 9 billion. Now, if we do a really great job on new vaccines, health care, reproductive health services, we could lower that by perhaps 10 or 15 percent."

If the hundreds of doctors and scientists predicting 100% death within three to five years for everyone taking the jab are right, then it's not a question of if, but when.

Time is of the essence. For all of us.

If you've already taken the jab, I strongly urge you get your soul in order. Actually, I advise everyone to do this, jabbed or not jabbed.

As I said earlier, I'm not entirely sure whether the vax and the vax passports are the Mark of the Beast, but there is an abundance of evidence that suggests either they are the Mark of the Beast or they are the frontrunners to it. To be safe, I think we all have to proceed as if they are.

A Gigantic Wake-Up Call from God

One thing I've learned from studying the cause and cure of all illness is that God sends us illness, accidents and other calamities as ways of getting our attention. He doesn't want to do it, but it's often the only thing that makes us stop and listen.

Most people refuse to listen to God unless and until they are facing some sort of crisis, usually a health crisis. If a crisis is the only way that God can get a person's attention, then what do you expect Him to do? Of course, He's going to send that person a crisis in order to get their attention and possibly save their soul.

With that thought in mind, look at what's happening on the world stage with hundreds of thousands of people suffering jab-related deaths and illnesses. It appears to be a giant wake-up call from God for all humanity. And if that is the case, it's even more confirmation that we are living in the end times.

The time to save your soul is now and the way to do it is to stop sinning and embrace the traditional (pre-Vatican II) Catholic Church.

When I say the Catholic Church, I mean the *true* Catholic Church, the pre-Vatican II Church that existed publicly up until the 1960s, and still exists today in small pockets.

What we see coming out of Rome today is not the Catholic Church. In fact, it's the complete opposite. It's the same with all of the schools, hospitals and church buildings today that call themselves Catholic. They are not Catholic and they do not represent the true Catholic Church. They represent a counterfeit church.

The true Catholic Church was infiltrated and subverted almost a century ago by the same Communists running the virus hoax.

Have you ever seen a counterfeit twenty dollar bill? At first glance, it looks just like the real thing. But take a closer look and it's clear that the bill is phony. And when you take a real close look, the fakery becomes so obvious that you wonder how you were ever fooled in the first place.

The same thing happens when you look at the counterfeit church that today pretends to be Catholic. Take a real close look and the fakery becomes so obvious that you wonder how anyone was ever fooled to begin with.

Similar to the virus hoax, in order to see the truth, it's necessary to leave emotions out of the equation and apply only facts, logic, and evidence. Most people are not able or willing to do that.

When it comes to the subject at hand–the Communist subversion and takeover of the Catholic Church and the creation of a counterfeit church–the deception is so huge, so monstrous, and so evil that hundreds of millions of people refuse to acknowledge it. They demonstrate the same mindset as those who were duped into believing the virus hoax. Many of them have been fooled into believing both, the virus hoax and the counterfeit church.

These folks are so frightened of the truth that the majority of them refuse to even look at the evidence. In fact, just mentioning this subject causes their hands to shake and the spittle to fly from their mouths. That's how frightened they are of the truth.

Saint Thomas Aquinas said, "The greatest charity one can do to another is to lead him to the truth."

As for me, I'm an evidence guy. I learned long ago that opinions are a cheap commodity, but evidence is something else. Evidence reigns supreme. I always follow the evidence, wherever it leads me, and let the chips fall where they may. Here's some evidence you might want to consider: the Catholic Church is the only religion in the world with tens of thousands of documented miracles.

From hard, physical evidence that you can see with your own eyes and touch with your own hands, such as the Shroud of Turin (the burial cloth of Jesus Christ) and the Blessed Virgin's miraculous imprint of herself on Juan Diego's tilma at Guadalupe, Mexico in 1530, to the 70,000 eye witnesses who were present for the Miracle of the Sun at Fatima, Portugal in 1917, the Catholic Church has it all:

saints whose bodies defy all science and physics by not decomposing after their death, miraculous healings, documented cases of saints raising the dead, documented cases of bilocation in which priests and mystics appear at two or more places at the same time, miraculous battlefield victories against incredible odds as high as 10,000 to 1, and on and on and on; literally tens of thousands of documented miracles within the true Catholic Church.

Meanwhile, all of the other religions of the world combined, numbering in the thousands, do not contain one single documented miracle among them. Not one. As I said, I side with the evidence.

Research the miracle of Our Lady of Guadalupe. Really research it. Do the same with the Miracle of the Sun, and then ask yourself how such supernatural miracles could have possibly occurred if the Catholic Church isn't the true church of Jesus Christ?

By research, I mean read reputable books on the subject, not the B.S. on Wikipedia or other internet "sources." The truth is out there, but you have to seek it.

Read These Books

I recommend you read the book *Outside the Catholic Church There is Absolutely No Salvation* by Brother Peter Dimond. You can find that book at several locations on the internet, and also at this specific website: www.MostHolyFamilyMonastery.com

If you can't afford to buy the book, which sells for around twenty bucks, then visit the website and read all of their free information. Watch their free videos. Immerse yourself in the truth.

Now if you're really courageous; if you're the absolute bravest of the brave, the strongest of the strong; afraid of no man and willing to do whatever it takes to achieve eternal glory, then read the book *Preparation for Death* by Saint Alphonsus Liguori.

I must warn you, it's not for the squeamish. You'll need the strength of Sampson to even begin reading it, and most people are too cowardly and too weak to do even that. It's that same cowardice and that same weakness that prevents the vast majority of men and women from resisting sin and leads to their being condemned to eternity burning in the fires of hell. All because they are too afraid to read a book or visit a website.

What about you?

Where do you stand?

You do want to go to Heaven, don't you?

In the old days when a ship sprung a leak or was caught in a storm and in danger of sinking, the passengers and crew would toss their belongings overboard in order to lighten the load and possibly save their lives. We have to apply the same tactic when it comes to saving our soul.

We must toss sinning overboard, along with any friend, family member, activity or situation which threatens our salvation. All of it has to go.

It a sacrifice, sure, but it's better to sacrifice now and ensure yourself eternal salvation than risk losing your soul.

I'll be right there with you, every step of the way.

Thank you very much for buying this book!

If you enjoyed it, please leave a review. Even a short, one-sentence review will help.

If you did not enjoy it, please email me with suggestions to improve the text: Mikestone114@yahoo.com

Mike Stone is the author of *Based*, a young adult novel about race, dating and growing up in America; *A New America*, a dark comedy set on Election Day 2016; and *Reversing the Side Effects of the COVID-19 Vaccine: How to Heal Yourself from Adverse Reactions to the Vaccine and Protect Yourself from Shedding*

Based

5 Stars! "Simply off the charts!"

5 Stars! "Couldn't put it down."

5 Stars! "Sharp and funny take on the upside down world we live in today."

A New America

On the most divisive day of the year, in the most racially-charged city in America, recently red-pilled movie producer John Duke is about to learn what political correctness really means: marching with the herd or losing everything, including his family.

5 Stars! "A well-written book of an America gone mad."

5 Stars! "More!! Great read!"

5 Stars! "An exciting well-written novel. The author uses no clichés, his descriptions are original, and as a whole the writing is very creative."

5 Stars! "A fast-paced exciting novel."

5 Stars! "Read it all in one sitting. Had to remind myself it's supposed to be fiction."

5 Stars! "I hope this book is read far and wide, because it is the truth."

5 Stars! "You would never see a book written like this in a mainstream publication."

Reversing the Side Effects of the COVID-19 Vaccine: How to Heal Yourself from Adverse Reactions to the Vaccine and Protect Yourself from Shedding

5 Stars! This is the fundamental work for all thinking beings.

5 Stars! "A whole lotta truth in this book."

Disclaimer

This work is for informational purposes only, and is not intended to diagnose or treat any disease. The author and publisher present the information, and the reader accepts it, with the understanding that everything done or tried as a result from reading this work is at the reader's own risk. The author and publisher have no liability or responsibility to any person or entity with respect to any loss, damage or injury caused, or alleged to be caused, directly or indirectly by the information contained in this book.

www.ingramcontent.com/pod-product-compliance
Lightning Source LLC
LaVergne TN
LVHW050942080826
845145LV00004B/1371

* 9 7 8 1 9 5 3 0 0 6 2 0 2 *